A Colour Guide to

The Assessment and Management of Leg Ulcers

Moya Morison, BSc, BA, MSc, RGN
Clinical Audit Co-ordinator
Stirling Royal Infirmary
Scotland

Wolfe Publishing Ltd

Published by
Wolfe Publishing Ltd
Brook House
2–16 Torrington Place
London WC1E 7LT

Printed by BPCC Hazells Ltd, Aylesbury, England

For full details of all Wolfe Nursing titles please write to Wolfe
Publishing Ltd, Brook House, 2–16 Torrington Place, London
WC1E 7LT, England.

British Library Cataloguing in Publication Data
   Morison, Moya J.
   A colour guide to the assessment and management
   of leg ulcers.
   (Clinical skills series)
   I. Title
   616.545

   ISBN 1 8700 6525 5

Contents

7056 — 616.545

Foreword

The need for attitudinal change towards leg ulcer disease was best underlined some years ago by the statement: heal the ulcer and the patient will die. How should such nihilism be tackled? First, we must understand the various mechanisms which are associated with leg ulcers and be able to discern that leg ulcers do not all have the same causes and are therefore unlikely to respond to the same treatment. Second, we must be able to diagnose the underlying nature of the leg ulcer accurately. Finally, we must apply logical, consistent and scientifically validated treatment that, above all, does no harm.

Over 80% of patients with leg ulcers never see a hospital clinic. Either they look after their own problems or they are cared for in the community. Community nurses will welcome a book that sets out recent advances in the understanding of the pathology of leg ulcers in a concise and clear way and gives clear direction on the assessment and the treatment of these patients.

Moya Morison has a background of science, teaching and nursing together with a long term interest in the management of wounds of all kinds. She is therefore ideally placed to write this book. After describing the magnitude of the problem in Chapter 1, attention is turned to the cause of leg ulcers. Chapter 2 provides a clear understanding of the causes of leg ulcers and aids in the development of skills that will help us recognize the important categories. There's more to patient assessment than meets the eye and it is well covered in Chapter 3. Treatment follows assessment. Chapter 4 crystallizes the previous three chapters and contains a particularly comprehensive section on local wound management. However, the importance of patient education and motivation is stressed in Chapter 5. The sad fact is that most ulcers recur; consequently Chapter 6 focuses on the prevention of recurrence and the beginning of a whole new phase of wound management.

Douglas R. Harper
Consultant Surgeon
Member of the Lothian and Forth Leg Ulcer Study
Falkirk and District Royal Infirmary
Scotland

Dedication

To Douglas and Barbara, with thanks for teaching me both the science and the art of healing leg ulcers.

Acknowledgements

This book has been made possible by the goodwill and encouragement of many people: my husband, Graeme, whose life has been so disrupted while helping with the preparation of the manuscript; my parents-in-law, Helen and Alastair, who dropped everything to type it; my parents, who ensured that I received the education to enable me to embark on the project; the staff of Stirling Royal Infirmary, who reviewed the work informally; and the patients from whom I have learned so much. My sincere thanks.

I would also like to thank the following companies and organizations who supplied illustrations used in this book:

Convatec (UK): *Figures 2.4, 2.7, 2.8, 4.5* and *4.13*.
Lederle Laboratories: *Figure 4.11*.
Medi (UK): *Figures 4.6* and *6.1*.
Perstorp Pharma: *Figure 4.9*.
Seton: *Figures 4.2* and *4.3*.
Smith & Nephew: *Figures 4.4, 4.10* and *4.14*.
Steriseal: *Figure 4.12*.
Stirling Royal Infirmary: *Figures 3.1, 3.2* and *4.16*.
Wolfe Publishing: *Figures 2.5, 4.1, 4.7, 4.8* and *4.15*.

1. *Epidemiology*

1.1   The size of the problem

Large scale studies, both in the UK and in Europe, suggest that about
1% of the population develop a leg ulcer at some point in their lives
(*Table 1.1*). One-fifth of these people have an open ulcer at any one time.

The incidence of leg ulceration rises with age. Over the age of 65,
women are at far higher risk of developing a leg ulcer than men. The
reasons for this are unclear but hormonal changes after the menopause
have been implicated.

Table 1.1 – Epidemiology of leg ulcers

Prevalence (open or healed)
Ten per thousand of the adult population, rising to 36
per thousand of the population over 65 years of age

Sex ratio	Male:Female
under 65	1:1
65–74	1:2.6
75–84	1:4.8
85+	1:10.3

Recurrence rates (%)	
1 episode	33
2–5 episodes	46
over 6 episodes	21

Healing rates (%)	
Time to heal	
up to 3 months	21
3 months to 1 year	29
1–5 years	40
over 5 years	10

Lothian and Forth Valley Leg Ulcer Study
(after Dale and Gibson, 1986)

Leg ulcers are notoriously slow to heal: 50% of ulcers are open for more than 1 year (Dale and Gibson, 1986; Cornwall *et al.*, 1986) and 10% are open for more than 5 years (*Table 1.1*). Chronic leg ulceration may plague some people for virtually the whole of their adult life. The recurrence rate for ulceration is also depressing, with about two-thirds of patients experiencing two or more episodes and 21% of patients more than six episodes. There is an old adage: 'Once an ulcer patient always a potential ulcer patient.' This is borne out by surveys that show that half the patients with an ulcer have a history of ulceration dating back at least 10 years (Callam *et al.*, 1987).

1.2 Who carries out the care?

In the UK there are very few specialist leg ulcer centres with outpatient clinics. The majority of patients are cared for in the community by district nurses, at general practitioners' surgeries, or by relatives, who may or may not be adequately instructed or supervised.

1.3 The cost of caring

Caring for leg ulcers can be very expensive. One survey found that 50% of patients with ulcers were having their dressings changed every 1–2 days, 16% twice a week and 26% once a week (Dale and Gibson, 1986).
  Determining the cost of treatment is difficult. Any costing should include:

● District nurses' time and travelling.
● Wound dressing materials, e.g. dressing packs, cleansing solutions, primary and secondary dressings and bandages.
● Hospitalization for: ulcers which will not heal; vascular surgery or skin grafting.

In 1990, staff at the Charing Cross Hospital's leg ulcer service estimated the annual cost of treating a leg ulcer to be between £2700 and £5200 per patient. It has been estimated that leg ulcers cost the National Health Service £300–600 million annually for the UK as a whole.

References

Callam, M.J., Harper, D.R., Dale, J.J., *et al.* (1987) Chronic ulcer of the leg: clinical history. *Br. Med. J.* **294**, 1389–1391.
Cornwall, J., Dore, C.J. and Lewis, J.D. (1986) Leg ulcers: epidemiology and aetiology. *Br. J. Surg.* **73**, 693–696.
Dale, J. and Gibson, B. (1986) The epidemiology of leg ulcers. *Professional Nurse* **1**(8), 215–216.

2. Causes of leg ulcers

2.1 Introduction

A number of factors, some acting together, can lead to the development of leg ulcers (*Table 2.1*). While a minor traumatic incident is usually the immediate cause of the ulcer, the underlying problem is generally vascular.

Table 2.1 – Causes of leg ulcers

A. Principal causes

1. *Chronic venous hypertension.* Usually due to incompetent valves in the deep and perforating veins.
2. *Arterial disease.* Atherosclerotic occlusion of large vessels or arteritis of small vessels, leading to tissue ischaemia.
3. *Combined venous hypertension and arterial disease.*

B. Unusual causes (less than 1% in total)

1. *Malignancy.* Squamous cell carcinoma, melanoma or basal cell carcinoma.
2. *Infection.* Tuberculosis, leprosy, syphilis, deep fungal infections (all rare causes in the UK but still seen in the tropics).
3. *Blood disorders.* Polycythaemia, haemoglobinopathies.
4. *Metabolic disorders.* Pyoderma gangrenosum, pretibial myxoedema.
5. *Lymphoedema.* Normally only associated with ulceration when venous hypertension is also present or following cellulitis.
6. *Trauma.* Usually the immediate cause of ulceration in most cases, and the primary cause in a few cases where there is no clinically significant underlying vascular problem.
7. *Iatrogenic.* Over-tight bandaging, or ill-fitting plaster cast.
8. *Self-inflicted.*

Over 70% of leg ulcers encountered in the UK are primarily the result of *chronic venous hypertension* (see Section 2.2; *Figure 2.3*). *Poor arterial blood supply* accounts for about 10% of leg ulcers (see Section 2.3; *Figure 2.6*), and a further 10–15% of ulcers are of *mixed arterial and venous origin.*

More unusual causes of ulceration, amounting to no more than 1% of the total, include malignancy, infection, lymphoedema, blood disorders and certain metabolic disorders. A few leg ulcers are primarily due to trauma, some are a secondary complication of treatment and an unknown proportion are self-inflicted.

Identifying the underlying cause of the ulcer has important implications for treatment. To understand the major causes of ulceration requires an understanding of the anatomy of the vascular system of the lower limb and the mechanics of its blood flow.

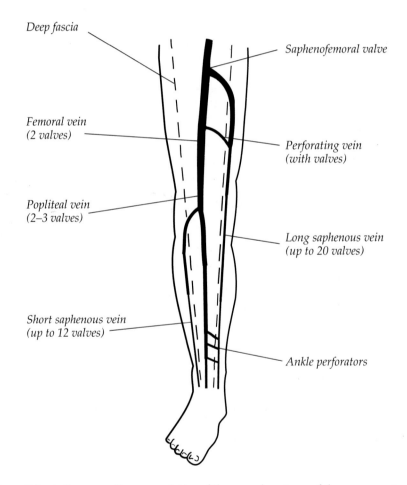

Figure 2.1. A diagrammatic representation of the normal anatomy of the venous system of the leg (based on Orr and McAvoy, 1987).

2.2 Venous ulcers

2.2.1 Anatomy of the venous system and mechanics of bloodflow

Both superficial and deep systems of veins are found in the leg (*Figure 2.1*). The superficial long and short saphenous veins are designed to carry blood under low pressure and have many valves to prevent back flow. They lie outside the deep fascia and drain into the deep vein system, which comprises the popliteal and femoral veins. The deep veins are designed to carry blood back to the heart under much higher pressure and they have fewer valves. The superficial and deep systems are connected by perforating veins which pass through the fascia. Blood is returned to the heart from the periphery, via the venous system, by a combination of mechanisms acting together; these include muscle contraction, capillary pressure and variations in intra-abdominal and intrathoracic pressure.

Active calf muscles, in their semi-rigid fascial envelope, act as a pump, forcing deep venous blood upwards towards the heart. When healthy and intact, the valves in the perforating veins prevent back flow of blood to the superficial system (*Figure 2.2a*). During periods of muscle relaxation blood flows from the superficial veins to an area of

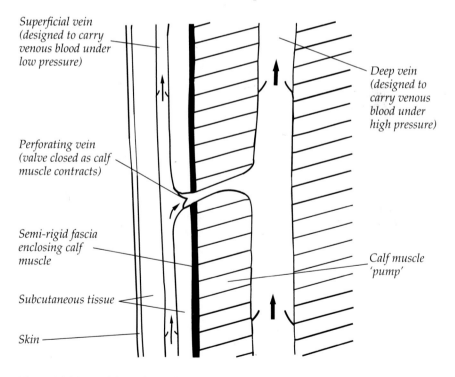

Figure 2.2(a). Healthy, intact valves prevent backflow of blood from the deep to the superficial veins.

5

temporarily lower pressure in the deep veins (beneath the closed valves), filling them, before the calf muscle pump acts again to force this blood centrally away from the extremities.

If the valves in the perforating veins become incompetent (*Figure 2.2b*), the back pressure is transmitted directly to the superficial venous system, damaging more distal valves and eventually leading to varicose veins. Damaged valves in the deep and perforating veins result in *chronic venous hypertension* in the lower limb, the high back pressure causing *venous stasis* and *oedema*.

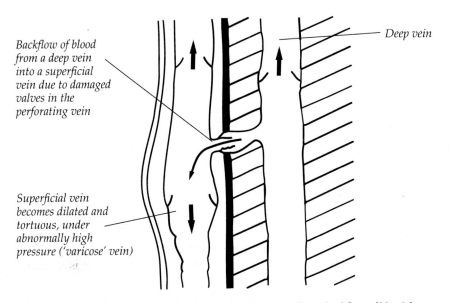

Backflow of blood from a deep vein into a superficial vein due to damaged valves in the perforating vein

Deep vein

Superficial vein becomes dilated and tortuous, under abnormally high pressure ('varicose' vein)

Figure 2.2(b). An incompetent valve in a perforating vein allows backflow of blood from the deep to the superficial venous system.

The role of the calf muscle pump in aiding venous return has been described. The ankle movement involved in walking is also important, as tensioning the Achilles tendon alternately stretches and relaxes the calf muscle, independently of calf muscle contraction, further aiding venous return. Another mechanism is involved in aiding venous return from the foot: emptying of the foot veins is facilitated by external pressure as the heel strikes the ground during walking (Gardner and Fox, 1986).

In patients who are 'off their feet' neither the foot pump nor the calf muscle pump can operate, and the efficiency of venous return is markedly impaired.

Some patients' mobility is limited by restricted ankle movement, as seen in people with, for example, extensive ulceration in the gaiter area, lipodermatosclerosis (hardening of the dermis and underlying subcutaneous fat) or with extensive fibrosis. Restricted ankle movement makes venous return of blood to the heart much less efficient.

2.2.2   Clinical signs of chronic venous hypertension
Some of the complications arising from chronic venous hypertension are summarized in *Figure 2.3* and described below.

Varicose veins   Varicose veins are a common problem, found in 10–20% of the adult population. People in occupations which involve prolonged standing in warm conditions, such as nurses, airline hostesses, teachers and storemen, are particularly at risk (*Table 2.2*).

Table 2.2 – Factors thought to predispose the development of varicose veins

1. *Family history.*
2. *Occupation:* those involving standing in warm conditions.
3. *Gender:* more common in women than men with increasing age.
4. *Pregnancy.*
5. *Low fibre diet.*
6. *Obesity.*

Varicose veins are a sign of chronic venous hypertension in the lower limb, which is usually due to damage to the valves in the leg veins. The damage may be congenital or acquired (*Table 2.3*). The result is that the superficial venous network is exposed to much higher pressures than normal (up to 90 mmHg instead of 30 mmHg). The superficial veins, especially the relatively thin-walled tributaries of the long and short saphenous veins, become dilated, lengthened and tortuous. About 3% of patients with varicose veins go on to develop leg ulcers.

Table 2.3 – Causes of varicose veins and raised venous pressure in the lower leg

1. *Primary*	● Due to congenital defect in the vein wall (collagen defect).
	● Due to valve cusps absent or abnormal.
2. *Secondary*	● *Obstructed venous return* due to pregnancy, pelvic tumours or ascites; leads to prolonged back pressure in the venous system and incompetent deep and perforating vein valves.
	● *Distortion of the valve cusps* caused by deep vein thrombosis (resulting, for example, from leg injury, prolonged immobility, pregnancy and surgery).

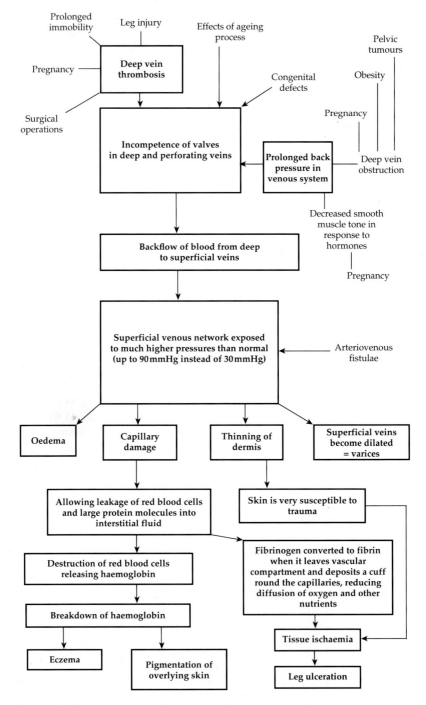

Figure 2.3. Venous ulcers: pathophysiology—a tentative model.

Staining of skin in the gaiter area Chronic venous hypertension leads to distension of the blood capillaries, with resulting damage to the endothelial walls and leakage of red blood cells and large protein molecules into the interstitial fluid (*Figure 2.3*). Destruction of the red blood cells releases breakdown products of haemoglobin, leading to pigmentation of the overlying skin (*Figure 2.4*).

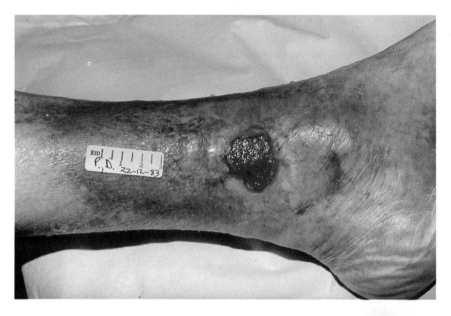

Figure 2.4. A venous ulcer.

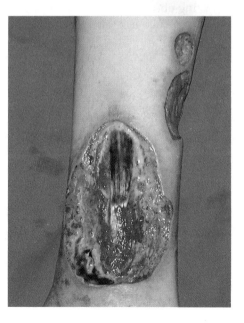

Figure 2.5. A deep arterial ulcer in a patient with rheumatoid arthritis, with exposed tendon and necrotic tissue visible. The underlying vascular problem is arteritis.

9

Ankle flare Chronic venous hypertension can cause distension of the tiny veins on the medial aspect of the foot. This is particularly noticeable where the valves in the perforating veins in the ankle and lower calf are incompetent, and is sometimes referred to as 'ankle flare' (*Figure 2.4*).

Atrophy of the skin Browse and Burnand (1982) have put forward the hypothesis that when blood capillaries are exposed to high pressures fibrinogen leaks out of damaged capillaries and is deposited round them as a fibrin cuff. This is thought to inhibit both the diffusion of oxygen and nutrients to surrounding tissues and the removal of metabolic waste products. Diffusion is further impaired by the presence of excess interstitial fluid in oedematous limbs.

Thinning of the dermis, associated with a poor blood supply, makes the skin very susceptible to trauma. Other trophic changes include stasis eczema and lipodermatosclerosis.

Eczema Wet or dry eczema is often associated with a poor peripheral blood supply and can be aggravated by a number of wound care products (see Section 4.5.3.6).

Lipodermatosclerosis 'Woody' induration of the tissues and fat necrosis is seen as an end-stage phenomenon. The leg often assumes the shape of an 'inverted champagne bottle', wide at the knee and very narrow at the ankle.

Ulceration is the end point of the trophic changes described above, affecting about 1% of the adult population and about 3% of people with varicose veins. It is often precipitated by a *minor traumatic event*, such as a knock while alighting from a car, which would not cause significant skin breakdown in a person with a healthy circulation in the leg.

2.3   Arterial ulcers

There are many causes of ischaemia in the lower leg, the most common being *atherosclerosis*. The coexisting atheroma and arteriosclerosis are degenerative changes often associated with advancing age. Other risk factors which can influence the severity of atherosclerosis include: *being of male sex*, *hypertension* and *smoking*.

Other causes of ischaemia include *rheumatoid arthritis* (*Figure 2.5*) and *diabetes mellitus*, which tend to affect smaller distal arteries, *Buerger's disease* and *Raynaud's disease*. Arterial embolism and trauma can cause acute ischaemia, which is potentially the most damaging (as well as life threatening), because the body has not had time to develop a collateral circulation to compensate.

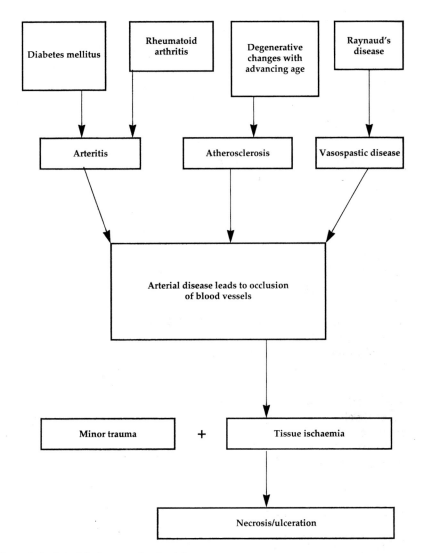

Figure 2.6. Arterial ulcers: pathophysiology.

The relationship between arterial disease and arterial ulcers is summarized in *Figure 2.6*. Tissue ischaemia resulting from a narrowing or distortion of arterioles predisposes to necrosis and ulceration following minor trauma. The skin surrounding the ulcer is often shiny, hair loss is common, but there is no brown staining in the gaiter area unless there are also venous problems (*Figure 2.7* and *Figure 2.8*).

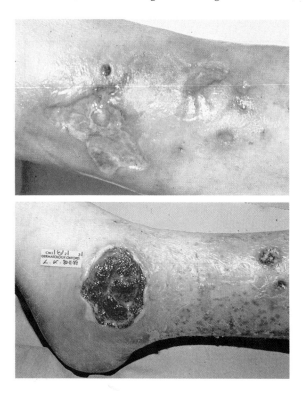

Figure 2.7. Superficial multiple ulcers in a diabetic patient.

Figure 2.8. An arterial ulcer on the lateral malleolus.

The significance of an arterial component in leg ulcer aetiology is being increasingly recognized. Both Cornwall *et al.* (1986) and Callam *et al.* (1987a) estimated that about 21% of patients presenting with leg ulcers have evidence of arterial insufficiency. This has very important implications for treatment (Callam *et al.*, 1987b). The accurate differential diagnosis of venous and arterial leg ulcers is therefore essential (see Chapter 3).

References

Browse, N.L. and Burnand, K.G. (1982) The cause of venous ulceration. *Lancet* **ii**, 243–245.

Callam, M.J., Harper, D. R., Dale, J.J. *et al.* (1987a) Arterial disease in chronic leg ulceration: an under-estimated hazard? Lothian and Forth Valley Leg Ulcer Study. *Br. Med. J.* **294**, 929–931.

Callam, M.J., Ruckley, C.V., Dale, J.J. *et al.* (1987b) Hazards of compression treatment of the leg: an estimate from Scottish surgeons. *Br. Med. J.* **295**, 1382.

Cornwall, J., Dore, C.J. and Lewis, J.D. (1986) Leg ulcers: epidemiology and aetiology. *Br. J. Surg.* **73**, 693–696.

Gardner, A.M.N. and Fox, R.H. (1986) The return of blood to the heart against the force of gravity. In Negus, D. and Jantet, G. (eds) *Phlebology '85*, pp. 65–67. Libbey, London.

Orr, M.M. and McAvoy, B.R. (1987) Varicose veins and their effects. In Fry, J. and Berry, H.E. (eds) *Surgical Problems in Clinical Practice*, pp. 111–122. Edward Arnold, London.

3. *Patient assessment*

3.1   Introduction

When a patient presents for the first time with a leg ulcer a general patient assessment is required to determine:

- The underlying *cause* of the ulcer.
- Any *local problems at the wound site* which may delay healing, such as infection, excess exudate or necrotic tissue.
- Other general *medical conditions* which may delay healing.
- The patient's *social circumstances* and the optimum setting for care.

3.2   Assessing the underlying cause of the ulcer

Unless the underlying cause of the ulcer is determined and, where possible corrected, delayed wound healing is inevitable. At worst, inappropriate treatment can lead to the necessity to amputate the limb.

Assessment of the patient's clinical signs and symptoms, past medical history and some simple investigations normally give sufficient information for the nurse to decide whether the patient is presenting with an ulcer due to:

- Chronic venous hypertension (70%).
- Arterial disease (about 10%).
- A combination of chronic venous hypertension and arterial disease (10–20%).
- Some other cause (about 1%).

If there is any doubt about the underlying aetiology of an ulcer, the nurse who is assessing a patient is strongly advised to refer the patient to a doctor, as soon as possible, to arrange for further tests.

3.2.1 *Clinical signs and symptoms*

The clinical signs and symptoms of venous and arterial disorders in the lower limb are summarized in *Tables 3.1* and *3.2*. An explanation of the underlying pathophysiology which gives rise to these signs and symptoms is given in Chapter 2, which discusses the mechanisms leading to ulceration.

Table 3.1 – Venous problems: clinical signs and symptoms

1. *Prominent superficial leg veins or symptoms of varicose veins*
    - *Aching* or *heaviness* in legs, generalized or localized.
    - Mild ankle *swelling*.
    - *Itching* over varices.
    - Symptoms due to thrombophlebitis, localized *pain, tenderness* and *redness*.

    Gentle exercise such as walking round the room or repeated heel raising helps to show distension of the veins
2. *Skin surrounding the ulcer*
    - *Ankle flare* distension of the tiny veins on the medial aspect of the foot below the malleolus.
    - *Pigmentation* 'staining' of the skin around the ulcer due to breakdown products of haemoglobin from extravasated red blood cells.
    - *Lipodermatosclerosis* hardening of dermis and underlying subcutaneous fat.
    - *Stasis eczema*.
    - *Atrophe blanche* ivory white skin stippled with red 'dots' of dilated capillary loops.
3. *Site of ulcer*
    - Frequently near the medial malleolus, sometimes near the lateral malleolus.
4. *Characteristics of the ulcer*
    - *Depth and shape* usually shallow, with flat margins; often an elongated oval in shape (see *Figure 2.4*).
    - *Pain* only painful if grossly infected and/or there is marked peripheral oedema.
    - *Changes over time* develop slowly if untreated unless seriously infected, e.g. with β-haemolytic streptococci.

Table 3.2 – Arterial problems: clinical signs and symptoms

1. *Whole leg/foot*
   Symptoms
   - *Intermittent claudication:* cramp-like pain in the muscles of the leg, brought on by walking a certain distance (depending partly on speed, gradient and patient's weight). The patient then has to stop and stand still to rest the ischaemic calf muscles.
   - *Ischaemic rest pain:* intractable constant ache felt in the foot, typically in the toes or heels overnight in bed. Usually relieved by dependency: hanging the leg over the bed or sleeping upright in a chair.

   Signs
   - Coldness of the foot (but not specific to ischaemia).
   - Loss of hair.
   - Atrophic, shiny skin.
   - Muscle wasting in calf or thigh.
   - Trophic changes in nails.
   - Poor tissue perfusion, e.g. colour takes more than 3s to return after blanching of toe-nail bed by applying direct pressure.
   - Colour changes foot/toes dusky pink when dependent, turning pale when raised above the heart.
   - Gangrene of toes.
   - Loss of pedal pulses.

2. *Site of ulcer*
   - Usually on the foot or lateral aspect of the leg but may occur anywhere on the limb, including near the medial malleolus (most common site for venous ulcers).

3. *Characteristics of the ulcer*
   - *Depth and shape:* often deep with loss of tissue exposing muscle and tendons, especially if the patient has rheumatoid arthritis; often irregular in shape and may be multiple small lesions, e.g. in diabetic patients (see *Figures 2.5* and *2.7*).
   - *Pain:* can be very painful.
   - *Changes over time:* rapid deterioration is characteristic.

3.2.2   Past medical history

Table 3.3 – Past medical history

---

1. *Indicators of possible venous problems*
   - *Previous thrombogenic events*
     Has the patient ever suffered from one or more of the following:
     > deep vein thrombosis
     > thrombophlebitis
     > leg or foot fracture
     in the affected limb?
   - *Varicose veins*
     Does the patient have prominent superficial leg veins, with signs of valve incompetence?
     Has the patient ever had any varicose vein surgery or sclerotherapy in the affected leg?
2. *Indicators of possible arterial problems*
   - *Generalized arterial disease*
     Are there any indicators of arterial disease such as:
     > previous myocardial infarction
     > angina
     > transient ischaemic attacks
     > intermittent claudication
     > cerebrovascular accident
     > diabetes mellitus
     > rheumatoid arthritis?

Table 3.3 summarizes the factors in a patient's past medical history which may throw some light on the underlying vascular problems which led to the development of the ulcer.

Chronic venous hypertension is suggested by a history of varicose veins with valve incompetence which may have been precipitated by any one or more of a number of thrombogenic events, e.g. leg fracture, immobility post surgery or during pregnancy (see *Figure 2.3*).

Callam *et al.* (1987) found that a history of stroke, transient ischaemic attacks, angina or myocardial infarction increased the probability of *arterial* impairment in the lower limb, and a history of intermittent claudication was almost invariably associated with poor peripheral perfusion.

3.2.3   Simple vascular assessment

In the past *the presence of palpable foot pulses* has been taken as a sign of unimpaired arterial circulation, and the *absence* of pulses as indicative of arterial impairment. This is not an entirely 'fail-safe' test. Oedema is a common problem in patients with venous ulcers and this can make pulses hard to feel.

A simple vascular assessment technique which can be readily carried out by nurses with a little training is the *resting pressure index (RPI) test*. This is a most important starting point in patient assessment and requires little practice to become proficient. It involves determining the ratio of ankle to brachial systolic pressures using a simple hand-held, battery operated Doppler ultrasound probe in place of a stethoscope. To overcome the effects of gravity, the patient should sit with the legs elevated on a stool for at least 20 min before the ankle systolic pressure is measured. During this time the patient's history can be taken and the brachial systolic pulse measured in the usual way. To assess the ankle systolic pressure the cuff is sited just above the malleolar area (above the ulcer) and the pressure measured using either the posterior tibial or dorsalis pedis pulse (*Figure 3.1* and *Figure 3.2*).

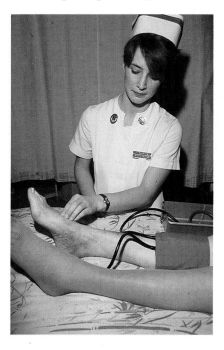 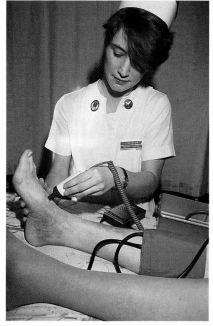

Figure 3.1. Finding the dorsalis pedis pulse by palpation.

Figure 3.2. The use of doppler ultrasound to measure the ankle systolic pressure.

$$\text{Resting pressure index (RPI)} = \frac{\text{ankle systolic pressure}}{\text{brachial systolic pressure}}$$

The RPI allows for individual variations in blood pressure and should normally be greater than 1.0. Patients with a ratio of 0.9–0.95 probably have some degree of arterial disease. If the RPI is less than 0.8 there is significant impairment in the arterial blood supply, which means that compression bandaging is contraindicated. A ratio of 0.5–0.75 is often associated with intermittent claudication, and <0.5 with ischaemic rest pain. A rapid referral to a doctor is advisable if the index is below 0.75.

A resting pressure index above 1.2 may be pathological, for instance in a patient with medial calcinosis. In diabetic patients a falsely high RPI may be obtained. **No graduated compression should be applied to a diabetic patient's leg, except under the closest medical supervision.** If there is any doubt about the significance of the RPI a doctor should be consulted for further advice.

3.2.4   Other investigations
Some further investigations can yield valuable results (*Table 3.4*).

Table 3.4 – Other simple investigations

1. *Urinalysis* particularly to detect undiagnosed diabetes, which is often associated with peripheral arterial problems.
2. *Blood tests* to test for rheumatoid and antinuclear factors which may indicate potential arteritis or autoimmune disorders; full blood count and estimation of haemoglobin levels.
3. *Patch testing for allergens*, e.g. lanolin and parabens, which are present in many commonly used wound care products.
4. *Tissue biopsy* if malignant changes are suspected.
5. *Wound swabs* to identify the causation and antibiotic sensitivity of any organisms causing clinical signs of infection.

3.2.5   Further vascular assessment methods

The physician may decide to request a more detailed vascular assessment, especially if localized occlusion of a blood vessel, which might be amenable to surgery, is suspected. Options include:

- Venography (ascending phlebography): this is useful for detecting acute thrombosis, chronic occlusion of the deep veins with the development of collateral circulation, and incompetent perforators.
- Arteriography: a very useful method of investigating the site and extent of arterial occlusion, which is essential before any arterial reconstruction can be considered.

Incompetent valves in the perforating veins and saphenofemoral and saphenopopliteal reflux can be demonstrated using portable Doppler ultrasound equipment (Ruckley, 1988). Such assessment requires considerable experience and is generally the province of the vascular surgeon. Other non-invasive vascular laboratory assessment techniques include foot volumetry to assess the efficiency of the foot and calf muscle pumps, plethysmography to measure ambulatory venous pressure (Norris et al., 1983), and ultrasound imaging, which allows direct imaging of the deep and superficial veins (Ruckley, 1988).

3.2.6 Mixed aetiology ulcers

Between 10% and 20% of leg ulcers do not fall neatly into either the venous or arterial categories. A patient's leg may show all the classic signs of chronic venous hypertension, but there may also be underlying arterial problems. The checklist in *Table 3.5* can be used to help to determine whether the ulcer is likely to be of venous, arterial or mixed aetiology.

Of leg ulcers, 1% are not due to vascular problems (see *Table 2.1*). If the wound has an unusual appearance, is refractory to healing or if the patient has recently arrived in the UK from abroad, a more unusual cause should be suspected.

If the nurse is unsure of the underlying cause of any ulcer she should refer the patient to a doctor for further assessment.

3.3   Assessing the ulcer

After assessing the underlying cause of the ulcer, assessment of the wound itself should be undertaken, as this may determine the method of wound cleansing and the most appropriate primary wound contact dressing.

To enable the effectiveness of treatment to be assessed it is helpful to *trace* the ulcer using an acetate sheet or transparent glove and a fine permanent marker pen. The tracing can be annotated with information such as the nature of the wound bed and wound margins, some indication of the depth of the wound, the date and the patient's name (*Figure 3.3*).

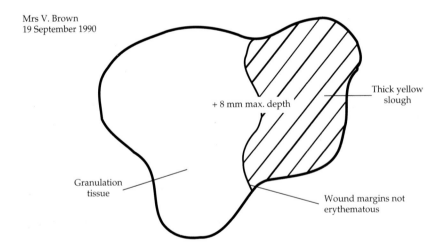

Mrs V. Brown
19 September 1990

Thick yellow slough

+ 8 mm max. depth

Granulation tissue

Wound margins not erythematous

Figure 3.3. Leg ulcer tracing.

Table 3.5 – Differential diagnosis of venous and arterial leg ulcers: some points to consider when assessing patients (tick boxes that apply to the patient; the pattern of ticks should give some indication of the underlying aetiology of the ulcer)

Indicators of venous problems

1. *Past medical history*
   - Has the patient ever suffered from any of the following: deep vein thrombosis, thrombophlebitis or leg/foot fracture in the affected limb? ☐
   - Has the patient ever had any varicose vein surgery or sclerotherapy in the affected limb? ☐

2. *Clinical signs and symptoms in the leg*
   - Prominent superficial leg veins. ☐☐
   - Brown pigmentation of the skin around and just above the ankle. ☐☐
   - Distension of the tiny veins in the medial aspect of the foot. ☐
   - Lipodermatosclerosis (hard 'woody' induration of the lower leg). ☐☐
   - Stasis eczema.
   - Atrophe blanche (skin thin, white and stippled with red dots).

3. *The ulcer*
   - Ulcer shallow, flat margins. ☐☐☐
   - Ulcer not painful (unless clinically infected).
   - Site of ulcer: near medial or lateral malleolus (but may be anywhere).

4. *Simple vascular assessment/tests*
   - Pedal pulses present. ☐☐
   - Resting pressure index (RPI) >0.9.

Indicators of arterial problems

1. *Past medical history*
   - Are there any indicators of generalized arterial disease, e.g. myocardial infarction, angina, transient ischaemic attacks, intermittent claudication, cerebrovascular accident, diabetes mellitus, rheumatoid arthritis? ☐

2. *Clinical signs and symptoms in the leg*
   - Intermittent claudication. ☐☐☐☐
   - Ischaemic rest pain.
   - Pain relief when the leg is lowered below heart level. ☐
   - Foot dusky pink when dependent, turning pale when elevated above the heart.
   - Poor tissue perfusion, e.g. colour takes more than 3 s to return after blanching of toe-nail bed by applying direct pressure. ☐
   - Loss of hair, atrophic shiny skin.

3. *The ulcer*
   - Ulcer deep, with loss of tissue exposing muscle and tendon. ☐
   - Ulcer very painful. ☐☐
   - Site of ulcer: on foot or lateral aspect of the leg (but may be anywhere).

4. *Simple vascular assessment/tests*
   - Pedal pulses absent or very faint indeed. ☐☐
   - Resting pressure index (RPI) < 0.9.

OPEN WOUND ASSESSMENT CHART

Type of wound (e.g. venous or arterial leg ulcer) ....

Location..

How long has wound been open?...

General patient factors which may delay healing (e.g. malnourished, diabetic, chronic infection)..

....

Allergies to wound care products ....

Previous treatments tried (comment on success/problems)

a. Débridement..

b. Primary dressings ....

....

....

TRACE THE WOUND EVERY TWO WEEKS, ANNOTATING TRACING WITH MAXIMUM DIMENSIONS (length, breadth), NATURE OF WOUND BED, ORIENTATION OF WOUND

All other parameters should be assessed at **every** dressing change and changes documented.

Wound factors/Date								
1. **NATURE OF WOUND BED** a. healthy granulation b. epithelialization c. sloughy d. hard black necrotic								
2. **EXUDATE** a. colour b. amount: heavy/moderate/ minimal/none								
3. **ODOUR** Offensive/some/none								
4. **PAIN (SITE)** Specify								
5. **PAIN (FREQUENCY)** Continuous/intermittent/ only at dressing changes/none								
6. **PAIN (SEVERITY)** Patient's score (0–10)								
7. **WOUND MARGIN** a. colour b. oedematous?								
8. **ERYTHEMA OF SURROUNDING SKIN** a. present b. max. distance from wound (mm)								
9. **GENERAL CONDITION OF SURROUNDING SKIN** (e.g. dry eczema)								
10. **INFECTION** a. suspected b. wound swab sent c. confirmed (specify organism)								

WOUND ASSESSED BY:

Figure 3.4. Open wound assessment chart.

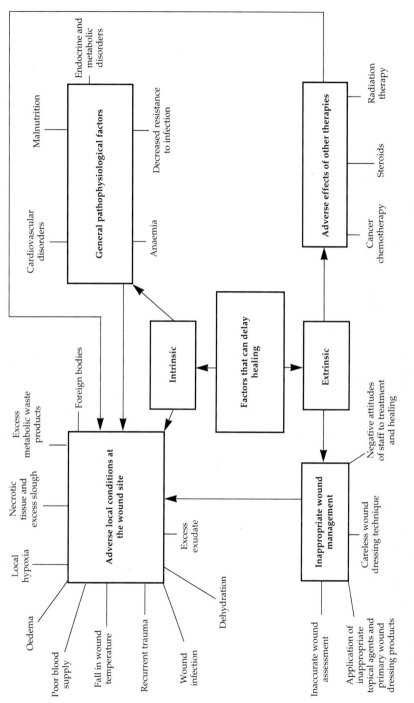

Figure 3.5. Factors causing delayed wound healing.

23

Offensive odour, the general condition of the surrounding skin, the nature and severity of pain at the wound site or elsewhere, the possibility of infection and whether or not a wound swab has been sent for culture and antibiotic sensitivity testing should also be noted, as should any previous allergies to wound care products.

Charting the healing of leg ulcers (*Figure 3.4*) is a very helpful aid to evaluating the effectiveness of local wound treatment. If a leg ulcer shows no signs of healing it may be because:

● The local problems at the wound site have not been dealt with appropriately.
● The underlying cause of the ulcer has not been identified and corrected.
● Some other patient factor is delaying healing.

3.4 Other factors that may affect healing

When taking the patient's history and carrying out an assessment of the patient's current general physical condition, it is worth noting any other factors that could delay wound healing (*Figure 3.5*), such as:

● Evidence of or suspected *malnutrition.*
● *Poor mobility*, of whatever cause, which may adversely affect the calf muscle pump and venous return.
● An *occupation* or activities that involve prolonged standing, especially in warm conditions.
● *Decreased resistance to infection*, for whatever cause.
● Poor *social* circumstances.

The patient's occupation and social circumstances should also be considered when deciding on the practical arrangements for managing the ulcer.

References

Callam, M.J., Harper, D.R., Dale, J.J. *et al.* (1987) Arterial disease in chronic leg ulceration: an under-estimated hazard? Lothian and Forth Valley Leg Ulcer Study. *Br. Med. J.* **294**, 929–931.

Norris, C.S., Beyreau, A. and Barnes, R.W. (1983) Quantitative photoplethysmography in chronic venous insufficiency: a new method of non-invasive estimation of ambulatory venous pressure. *Surgery* **94**, 758–764.

Ruckley, C.V. (1988) *A Colour Atlas of Surgical Management of Venous Disease*, p. 30. Wolfe Medical Publications, London.

4. Treatment options

4.1 Priorities in leg ulcer management

Having assessed the patient, and identified the underlying cause of the ulcer and any local problems at the wound site, the next step is to plan appropriate care. The main priorities are:

- To *correct* the underlying cause of the ulcer (this normally means improving the patient's venous and/or arterial circulation in the affected limb).
- To *create* the optimum local environment at the wound site.
- To *improve* all the wider factors that might delay healing (especially poor mobility, malnutrition and psychosocial issues).
- To *prevent* complications (such as wound infection or tissue damage due to overtight bandaging).
- To *maintain* healed tissue.

The principles behind the management of venous, arterial and mixed aetiology ulcers are now described, with the emphasis on correcting the underlying cause of the ulcer. Creating the optimum local environment for healing is discussed in Section 4.5 and ways of correcting or alleviating the effects of general patient factors that can delay healing are discussed in Section 4.6.

4.2 Management of venous ulcers

4.2.1 Introduction

The main cause of venous ulceration is chronic venous hypertension, with very high pressures being exerted on the superficial system, usually due to incompetent valves in the deep or perforating veins (see Chapter 2). The primary aims of venous ulcer management are therefore:

- To *reduce* the pressure on the superficial venous system.
- To *aid* venous return of blood to the heart, by increasing the velocity of flow in the deep veins.
- To *discourage* oedema by reducing the pressure difference between the capillaries and the tissues.

The best way of achieving these aims is to apply *graduated compression* from the base of the toes to the knee. Methods of achieving graduated compression include:

- Bandages (e.g. Blue Line, Setopress, Veinopress, Elastocrepe).
- Shaped elasticated tubular bandages (e.g. Tubigrip).
- Compression stockings (e.g. Venosan, Sigvaris, Jobst, Medi (UK)).

Each method has advantages and disadvantages, as indicated in *Table 4.1.*

4.2.2 *Characteristics of compression bandages*
There are basically two types of compression bandage:

- Those containing an *elastomer*, such as rubber or Lycra, as in Blue Line, Elset and Tensopress.
- Those *without elastomer*, which rely on crimped cotton, wool, or rayon threads for their extensibility, such as Elastocrepe and all types of crepe bandage.

Elasticity The elasticity of the bandage determines:

- How much tension is necessary to achieve the required pressure.
- How well the bandage will maintain this pressure.
- Its conformability to the awkward contours of foot, ankle and leg.

Pressure Some of the factors affecting the pressure that can be achieved under a bandage are given in the following equation:

$$P \text{ is proportional to } \frac{N \times T}{C \times W}$$

where P is the pressure exerted by the bandage;
       N is the number of layers of bandage;
       T is the bandage tension;
       C is the circumference of the limb;
       W is the bandage width.

As can be seen from the equation, the more layers that are applied to the leg the higher the pressure obtainable.

Table 4.1 – Methods of achieving graduated compression

Method	Advantages	Disadvantages
1. Bandages	a. Can be left in situ for up to a week in the absence of excess exudate except for highest compression bandages, e.g. Blue Line. b. By varying the tension under which the bandage is applied the pressure can be varied to suit individual needs and tolerances. c. A range of bandages is available in the community. d. Relatively low initial cost.	a. Excessively high pressures can be obtained with the heavy compression bandages, especially on thin legs and over bony prominences. b. Not cosmetically acceptable to many, leading to low compliance. c. Uncomfortable in hot weather. d. May require patient to purchase a larger size of shoe to accommodate bandage. e. Some prone to slip, leading to tight bands.
2. Shaped elasticated tubular bandages	a. Two layers toe to knee useful in patients who cannot tolerate an elastic compression bandage. b. Can help to reduce bandage slippage when used over a medium–light compression bandage.	a. Not currently available in the community. b. Only slightly increases the pressures obtained when applied over a bandage; little sustained compression achieved when applied alone.
3. Elastic compression stockings	a. Pressure profiles of stockings are tested and known. b. A range of compression profiles is available to meet individual needs. c. Much safer than inappropriately applied heavy compression bandages. d. Cosmetically acceptable. e. Useful in preventing recurrence of ulceration.	a. Require proper fitting for length, ankle and calf size. b. Initial cost is high, but compares well with the cost of elastic compression bandages over 6 months. c. Difficult for patients with restricted movement to apply themselves. d. Compliance rate variable; high compression stockings often poorly tolerated by the elderly but well liked by younger patients who are more mobile.

Tension The bandage tension is proportional to:

● The *elasticity* of the bandage.
● How much the bandage is *stretched* when it is applied.
● How many times the bandage has been *washed*.
● How *long* the bandage has been in place.

Limb circumference The circumference of the limb also affects sub-bandage pressure. As the pressure exerted by the bandage is *inversely* proportional to the circumference of the leg the thinner the leg the higher the pressures obtainable. *Dangerously high pressures* can be achieved with very heavy compression bandages in frail elderly patients with thin legs, especially over bony prominences such as the malleolus and tibia, and over the tendinous prominences around the ankle (*Figure 4.1*). Conversely, it is difficult to achieve high compression on a wide diameter leg. When seeking to aid venous return, graduated compression is required, with the highest pressure at the ankle (30–40 mmHg), gradually decreasing to about 50% of this pressure just below the knee. Since most legs are considerably narrower at the ankle than at the knee, graduated compression is *automatically* achieved if the bandage is applied at the *same tension* all the way up the leg.

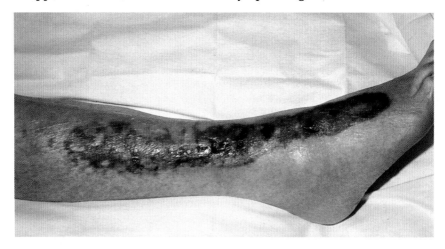

Figure 4.1. A bandage-induced ulcer which led to amputation.

The advantages and disadvantages of a range of compression bandages are given in *Table 4.2*. As new products for community use are regularly being added to the Drug Tariff, it is advisable to check which bandages are currently available.

4.2.3 Applying the bandage

It is helpful to place the patient's leg, with the foot at right angles, on a stool and at a height which is comfortable for the nurse to work at. All the materials required should be arranged so that they are within easy reach.

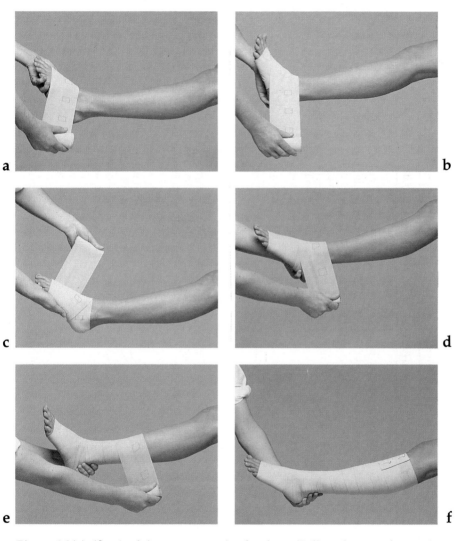

a
b
c
d
e
f

Figure 4.2(a)–(f). Applying a compression bandage. (Follow the manufacturer's instructions on precise method of application and the bandage tension required.)

Table 4.2 – Advantages and disadvantages of a number of commonly used compression and support bandages

Type of bandage	Examples (Manufacturer)	Advantages	Disadvantages
1. *Non-adhesive extensible bandages* Very high compression	Blue Line (Seton); Elastoweb (Smith & Nephew)	a. High pressures obtainable, suitable for counteracting venous stasis in the lower limb for active patients with venous ulcers (RPI $\geq$ 0.9 and preferably $\geq$ 1.0). b. Can be washed and reused.	a. High risk of tissue necrosis over bony prominences if inexpertly applied, especially to a thin leg. b. Must be taken off at night and reapplied in the morning, therefore only suitable for patients who can apply the bandage themselves. c. Cosmetically unacceptable to some patients.
Medium–high compression	Tensopress (Smith & Nephew); Veinopress (Steriseal); Setopress (Seton)	a. Good compression, well sustained, suitable for patients with venous ulcers (RPI $\geq$ 0.9). b. Less risk of pressure necrosis than with very high compression bandages. c. Can be worn continuously for up to one week. d. Comfortable and conformable. e. Can be washed and reused.	a. High pressures can be obtained over thin legs, therefore potentially hazardous if inexpertly applied.
Light compression/light support	Elastocrepe (Smith & Nephew)	a. Useful over paste bandages; increasing pressure achieved and pressure maintained over time (RPI $\geq$ 0.8).	a. Low pressures obtained; used alone it only gives light support. b. A single wash reduces

Type	Advantages / Uses	Disadvantages / Cautions
	b. Performance improved when covered with shaped elasticated tubular bandage which helps to prevent bandage slippage.	pressures obtained by about 20%. c. Bandage slippage can occur.
Light support only Crepe (Many manufacturers)	Only useful for: a. Holding dressings in place. b. As one of several layers in a multilayer bandage in treatment of venous ulcers. c. For light support of minor strains and sprains.	a. Pressures obtained are too low to be effective in management of venous ulcers. b. 40–60% of bandage tension (and hence pressure) lost in first 20 min after application.
2. *Cohesive extensible bandages* Cohesive bandages Tensoplus forte (Smith & Nephew); Coban (3M); Secure forte (Johnson & Johnson); Lestreflex (Seton)	a. Adhere to themselves, preventing slippage, therefore useful over non-adhesive bandages such as Elastocrepe, and over paste bandages. b. Compression well sustained. Suitable for patients with an RPI ≥ 0.85–0.9.	a. Can be hazardous in inexperienced hands as can cause tight bands round ankle and damage to tendons if wrongly applied.
3. *Hydrocolloid adhesive compression bandages* Hydrocolloid compression bandage Granuflex adhesive compression bandage (Convatec)	a. Good compression, well maintained (RPI > 0.8). b. Comfortable and conformable. c. Hydrocolloid can greatly improve condition of skin surrounding ulcers. d. Little slippage.	a. Not recommended for very fragile skin or where there is extensive wet eczema.

When applying any sort of compression to the lower leg it is important to include the *base of the toes* and to apply the bandage to just below the knee. Graduated compression can be obtained by applying the bandage *at the same tension* all the way up the leg, after suitably padding bony prominences. *Figure 4.2* shows how the bandage should be applied, beginning with the base of the toes, incorporating the heel and filling in under the foot before spiralling up the leg. Extra pressure can be achieved at the ankle by beginning the bandaging with a locking turn. This is particularly important when applying the lighter compression bandages, such as Elastocrepe, if they are to maintain reasonable pressures for several days.

Multi-layer bandaging Applying more than one layer of bandage can help to achieve good compression, even when only medium to low compression bandages are available. A layer of Velband (Johnson & Johnson) or Soffban (Smith & Nephew) is applied up to the knee, starting at the ankle to prevent excessive bulk over the foot. An Elastocrepe bandage is applied from the base of the toes to the knee, and this can be prevented from slipping by applying an outer layer of shaped elasticated tubular bandage. The size of the bandage required should be determined by measuring the circumference of the ankle and calf *after* the other layers have been applied. Any surplus should be cut off at the knee to prevent a garter effect from hindering venous return.

Another effective multi-layer regimen, developed at Charing Cross Hospital, London, is: Velband/Crepe/Elset/Coban. The Coban is a relatively inelastic cohesive bandage (*Table 4.2*) against which the calf muscle pump can act, aiding venous return.

Whichever bandaging regimen is used, care should be taken to overlap bandages evenly to prevent tight bands over bony prominences. Where bandages overlap, the pressure is higher than where there is a single layer of bandage. It is therefore important that each turn of the bandage overlaps its predecessor by half the bandage width to give an even pressure gradient. When the bandage is removed no deep grooves or indentations should be seen. Bandage damage can precipitate amputation, especially in ischaemic limbs where compression is contraindicated.

It is well worth practising bandaging technique on a friend before applying bandages to patients! One method of gaining a feeling for the pressures to be obtained is to inflate a sphygmomanometer cuff round the ankle to 40 mmHg and then move it up to the upper calf and inflate it to 20 mmHg. The cuff should feel pleasantly firm and supportive but not too tight.

Some bandages (e.g. Setopress) now include a simple visual guide to facilitate application of the bandage at the correct extension (*Figure 4.3*).

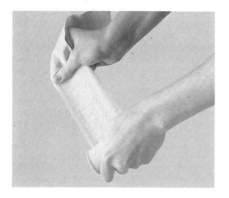 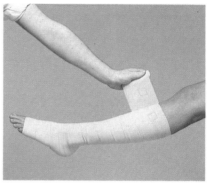

Figure 4.3(a). A simple visual guide to correct extension. The yellow rectangles become squares when the correct extension is reached.

Figure 4.3(b). The squares are covered over by the overlapping bandage.

Paste bandages For some patients with chronic skin disorders a paste bandage may be indicated (*Table 4.3, Figure 4.4*). Several layers are applied over the ulcerated area and the paste bandage is folded back over itself, over the bony prominences to prevent excessive pressure here and to allow the leg room to expand should it become oedematous (as may happen in hot weather or if the patient stands in one place for too long).

A double layer of tube gauze can be applied over the paste bandage before continuing with the multi-layer principle, e.g. Velband/Tensopress/shaped Tubigrip. Paste bandages are soothing and can rehydrate the skin surrounding the ulcer. Unfortunately, they contain ointment bases and preservatives that lead to sensitivity reactions in some patients (see Section 4.5.3.6).

Figure 4.4. A paste bandage being applied.

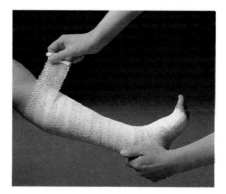

Table 4.3 – Paste bandages

Principal constituents	Proprietary name	Manufacturer	Indications
1. Zinc paste	Viscopaste PB7 Zincaband	Smith & Nephew Seton	General purpose treatment for leg ulcers, venous stasis eczema and chronic dermatitis. Soothing. Sensitivity reactions relatively infrequent.
2. Zinc paste and calamine	Calaband	Seton	Emollient properties, soothing and hydrating for dry, scaly lesions surrounding leg ulcers. Can be applied over ulcer itself.
3. Zinc paste and ichthammol	Ichthopaste	Smith & Nephew	Wet ulcers surrounded by sensitive skin. Soothing and mildly keratolytic. Ichthammol has a milder action than coal tar and is useful in less acute forms of eczema.
4. Zinc paste and coal tar	Coltapaste Tarband	Smith & Nephew Seton	Dry, itchy eczema where the skin surface has not broken down. Coal tar relieves itching and has keratolytic properties.

Hydrocolloid adhesive compression bandage A very interesting alternative to paste bandages is the *hydrocolloid adhesive compression bandage (HACB)* made by Convatec. This medium–high compression bandage (see *Table 4.2*) can be applied direct to the skin, with a hydrocolloid wafer dressing over the ulcer itself. The hydrocolloid in the bandage helps to rehydrate dry eczematous skin over the whole leg (Clay and Cherry, 1990) (*Figure 4.5*) and patients find it comfortable and conformable. There is minimum slippage of the bandage, which maintains good pressures for many days (Sockalingham *et al.*, 1990). The bandage is contraindicated, however, in patients with very fragile, paper-thin skin.

4.2.4 Compression stockings

Compression stockings have a number of advantages over bandages (see *Table 4.1*). They are a safe alternative, provided that the patient has been properly measured for them, and they are more cosmetically acceptable to many people. They are not, however, particularly easy to put on, but this problem can be overcome for many patients by supplying them with a dressing aid (*Figure 4.6*). Full length stockings are only required in a few instances, when treating patients with severe post-phlebitic syndrome, or lymphoedema with swelling in the thigh. Generally, below-knee stockings are all that is required, and as they are easier to apply than full length hosiery, compliance is likely to be better.

Compression stockings give graduated compression, with the greatest pressure exerted at the ankle, and are graded into three classes (Dale and Gibson, 1990):

Class I: Light compression, used to treat mild varicose veins.
Class II: Medium compression, for more serious varicosities, venous ulceration and venous ulcer prevention in patients with thin legs.
Class III: Heavy compression, for severe chronic venous hypertension, severe varicose veins and ulcer prevention and treatment in patients with large diameter legs.

4.2.5 Intermittent compression therapy

Pneumatic intermittent compression therapy can be helpful in reducing oedema and aiding venous return in hospitalized patients, but has been found to be less successful in patients living at home, as many patients are wary of the apparatus and are disinclined to use it (Hazarika and Wright, 1981).

4.2.6 Precautions when applying compression

Before any treatment is begun a full assessment of the patient should be carried out (see Chapter 3) to eliminate the possibility that the patient also has an arterial problem, with poor peripheral perfusion in the affected leg. Graduated compression should *not* be applied if:

● The resting pressure index is less than 0.8.
● The leg is oedematous.

The oedema must *not* be reduced by applying a compression bandage, as this could lead to extensive tissue damage. Limb elevation or bed rest may be required in severe cases (see Section 4.6.3.).
If in doubt consult the patient's doctor *before* applying compression.
Local wound management is discussed in Section 4.5.3.

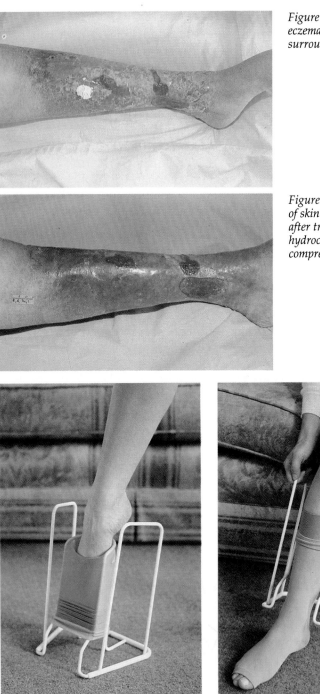

Figure 4.5(a). Dry eczematous skin surrounding an ulcer.

Figure 4.5(b). Rehydration of skin surrounding ulcer after treatment with a hydrocolloid adhesive compression bandage.

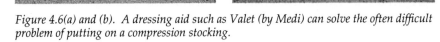

Figure 4.6(a) and (b). A dressing aid such as Valet (by Medi) can solve the often difficult problem of putting on a compression stocking.

4.3 Management of arterial ulcers

The prognosis for an elderly patient with an arterial ulcer is much less hopeful than that for a patient with a venous ulcer, properly treated, unless the underlying arterial problem is relatively local and is amenable to surgery. Where there are generalized arterial problems, such as arteritis, associated with rheumatoid arthritis, or microangiopathy, associated with diabetes mellitus, the treatment will be the doctor's responsibility. Vasodilator drugs are of questionable benefit, and even symptomatic relief of the effects of ischaemia is hard to achieve in some patients. The nurse's responsibility will be confined to symptom relief, local wound management (see Section 4.5.3) and patient education.

Patients should be encouraged to mobilize to the limit of their capabilities, to avoid smoking, to keep warm, to reduce weight, where this is a problem, and to eat a nutritious diet (see Section 4.6).

Compression bandaging should *not* be applied as severe damage to the leg can result (*Figure 4.7*) (see also *Figure 4.1*).

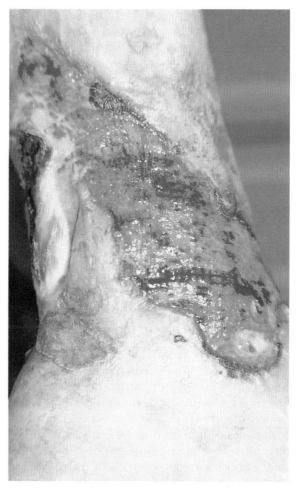

Figure 4.7. A deep arterial ulcer, with exposure of the Achilles tendon, which developed from a minor skin lesion, following application of an elastic bandage.

4.4　Management of mixed aetiology ulcers

Where the underlying cause of the ulcer appears to be a *combination* of chronic venous hypertension and poor peripheral arterial circulation, it is the degree of *arterial* insufficiency which will determine whether or not it is safe to apply compression. If the resting pressure index (RPI) is *less than 0.8 no compression* should be applied. If the RPI is 0.8–0.9 the patient may only tolerate light compression, such as a double layer of shaped elasticated tubular bandage (e.g. shaped Tubigrip) or a paste bandage with a light support bandage (see *Table 4.2*).

4.5　Creating the optimum local environment for healing

4.5.1　*Introduction*

Correcting the *underlying cause* of an ulcer, where possible, is the first principle of leg ulcer management but at the same time it is important to create the optimum conditions at the *wound site* to promote healing.

Adverse local conditions at the wound site that can delay healing are summarized in *Figure 3.5*, and include clinical infection, necrotic tissue, excess slough, excess exudate and dehydration. Priorities in wound management and the selection of the most appropriate primary wound dressing to overcome these problems are discussed in Section 4.5.3 and are reviewed in depth by Morison (1991). The use of ultrasound to stimulate healing is briefly mentioned in Section 4.5.4 and skin grafting is mentioned in Section 4.5.5.

Creating the optimum local environment for healing begins with cleansing the whole leg (Section 4.5.2).

4.5.2　*Cleansing the leg*

Before applying any kind of dressing to an ulcer it is important to render the whole of the lower leg 'socially clean'. One way to do this is to immerse the leg in a deep plastic bowl, lined with a disposable polythene bag and half filled with lukewarm tapwater. This helps to remove debris from the ulcer and the surrounding skin, and is comforting for the patient, especially if the leg has been encased in a multi-layer bandage regimen for the previous week. The leg can be gently dried with soft disposable paper and the bowl surface disinfected in accordance with the local infection control policy.

If the leg is known to be clinically infected by a virulent micro-organism, reversion to an aseptic technique for wound toilet is desirable, in the short term, to reduce both the risk of contaminating the physical environment and the risk of cross-infection.

The ulcer can then be traced (see *Figure 3.3*) before a dressing is applied.

4.5.3   Local wound management

4.5.3.1   Treating clinical infection   Chronic open wounds can be heavily *colonized* by micro-organisms, including many potential pathogens, without showing any adverse tissue response (Eriksson *et al.*, 1984). A number of studies have shown that the presence of colonizing micro-organisms does not delay healing. Indeed, delayed healing is *more* likely if aggressive measures are taken to attempt to keep a chronic wound 'bacteria free'. A wound swab should therefore only be sent to the bacteriology department for culture and antibiotic sensitivity testing if the wound shows *clinical signs and symptoms of infection,* such as excess, malodorous exudate, erythema of the wound margins, local pain and local oedema.

If cellulitis is present (*Figure 4.8*), the doctor may prescribe a *systemic antibiotic*. If a very virulent organism is isolated from a grossly infected open ulcer, with extensive tissue damage, in an immunocompromised patient, the use of a *topical antiseptic* such as povidone iodine may also be indicated (*Figure 4.9*). In cases of severe anaerobic infection the use of a hydrogel containing Metronidazole should be considered.

There is some evidence that the injudicious long-term use of topical antiseptics on chronic wounds can actually *delay* healing. The case against the use of hypochlorites, and other chlorine-releasing solutions such as Eusol, is strong (Brennan *et al.*, 1986; Leaper and Simpson, 1986), although it must be said that most of the studies have been done in animal models and *in vitro* rather than in humans. The uses and potential pitfalls of a number of popular cleansing agents and antiseptics are reviewed by Morison (1990).

A 'biological' alternative to the use of antiseptics in the local treatment of all but the most serious wound infections is to use an *enzyme based preparation,* e.g. Varidase, which breaks down the *waste products* of infection, such as pus and slough, and creates a clean wound bed. The balance is then tipped in favour of the body's own defence mechanisms and the arrested healing processes can recommence.

4.5.3.2   Removing necrotic tissue   The presence of dead or devitalized tissue in the wound bed delays healing and makes clinical infection more likely. The best method for treating this problem depends upon the nature of the necrotic tissue and the degree of debility of the patient. The necrotic tissue may be present in several forms such as hard black eschar and as slough.

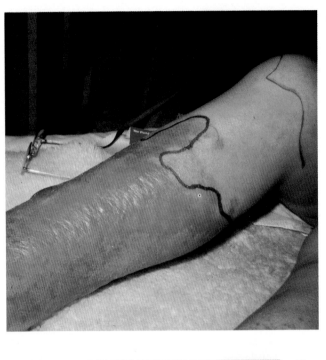

Figure 4.8.
Cellulitis.

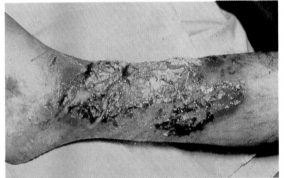

Figure 4.9(a). A grossly
infected leg ulcer, with
extensive necrotic tissue.

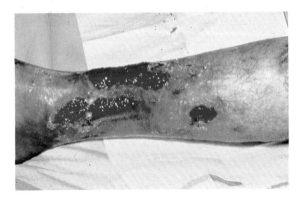

Figure 4.9(b). The same
ulcer after treatment of the
patient with a systemic
antibiotic and the local
application of Iodosorb
ointment.

Figure 4.10. Scherisorb gel being applied to a necrotic wound.

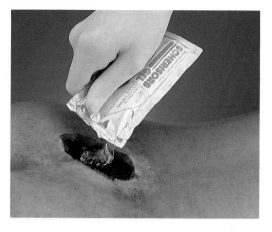

Figure 4.11(a). An extensive, necrotic ulcer in an elderly diabetic patient.

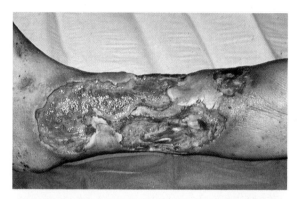

Figure 4.11(b). The same ulcer 7 days after débridement with an enzymatic preparation (Varidase).

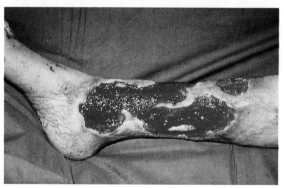

The main treatment options are:

- *Surgical débridement*. This is the quickest method and results in a wound bed of healthy tissue. It can sometimes be performed under a local anaesthetic but may not be suitable for severely debilitated patients.
- *Hydrocolloid dressing* (e.g. Granuflex) or a *hydrogel* (e.g. Scherisorb gel, *Figure 4.10*). These dressings help to create a local environment which encourages the body's natural débridement processes.
- *Enzymatic treatment* (e.g. Varidase, *Figure 4.11*). This can be applied to scored dry black eschar or to soft necrotic tissue in a gel form, with a secondary dressing. It can also be injected under hard black eschar but, as this is potentially hazardous if the solution is inadvertently injected into the systemic circulation, the manufacturer's instructions should be very strictly adhered to if this method is used.

Whichever method of débridement is finally selected **the manufacturer's recommendations should be consulted** concerning methods of application and removal, precautions and any contraindications.

The *hypochlorites* have been used in the past as débriding agents for treatment of soft necrotic tissue such as thick slough. However, they are quickly deactivated by body fluids and by the very waste products that they are likely to encounter, such as pus. Their use is *not recommended*, especially as there are much safer and more effective alternatives available today.

4.5.3.3 Managing malodorous ulcers   Heavily infected leg ulcers can be very malodorous. This can be distressing for the patient, leading to self-imposed social isolation, loss of appetite and depression. Treating the infection that leads to the malodorous exudate is important (see Section 4.5.3.1). The odour itself can be controlled in the short term by the use of an activated charcoal dressing, such as Actisorb Plus. Wherever possible, dressings and bandages should be changed before 'strike through' of exudate has occurred. This reduces both the risk of bacterial contamination through the wet dressing, and the risk of the wound drying out and the dressing adhering.

4.5.3.4 Dressings for clean, deep ulcers   Although they often have a large surface area, most venous ulcers tend to be shallow. Arterial ulcers, however, can rapidly deteriorate into deep wounds, with tissue loss involving muscle and exposing bone and tendon (see *Figure 2.5*). A very gentle treatment method is required, causing minimum trauma to the tissues as well as keeping the wound moist and thus reducing pain.

Methods for dressing clean, deep ulcers producing some exudate include:

- *Alginate dressings* (e.g. Sorbsan, *Figure 4.12*; and Kaltostat). These biodegradable dressings absorb excess exudate and encourage granulation.
- *Hydrocolloid wafer* (e.g. Granuflex or Granuflex E, *Figure 4.13*). Hydro-colloid paste can be gently applied to awkwardly shaped cavities and covered with a hydrocolloid wafer. Unless levels of exudate are very heavy, this regimen can usually be left in place for several days. The environment created under the dressing promotes new blood capillary formation, granulation and epithelialization.
- *Hydrogel* (e.g. Scherisorb gel). This creates a moist environment for healing. It must be covered by a secondary dressing.
- *Polyurethane foam sheet* (e.g. Allevyn, *Figure 4.14*). For relatively shallow, medium to heavily exudating ulcers.

If a wound is producing *copious volumes of exudate*, attempting to control this with a dressing is not enough. The skin surrounding the ulcer quickly becomes macerated, especially at the lower border, and strike through of exudate increases the risk of wound infection. The oedema should be reduced, as described in Section 4.6.3, and then the levels of exudate will lessen until a stage is reached when weekly dressing changes are sufficient. In the meantime, extra absorbent padding can be applied over the primary dressing and under the bandages.

4.5.3.5 Dressings for clean, shallow ulcers There are a number of primary dressings suitable for dressing clean, shallow leg ulcers, whether they are venous or arterial in origin:

- *Hydrocolloid wafer* (e.g. Granuflex). This has many of the charac-teristics of the ideal dressing. Not only does it provide a moist environment for healing which protects the underlying tissues from dehydration, but also it helps to protect against mechanical trauma and contamination by micro-organisms, as well as stimulating the formation of granulation tissue.
- *Simple low-adherence dressing* (e.g. Tricotex or NA + Dressing). Suitable as a primary wound contact layer in venous ulcers where an absorbent secondary layer is applied beneath the compression band-age regimen.
- *Paraffin tulle dressing* (e.g. Jelonet or Unitulle). As for simple low-adherence dressing (above).
- *Polyurethane foam dressing* (e.g. Lyofoam or Allevyn, see *Figure 4.14*). Use if the wound is producing medium to high volumes of exudate. The volume of exudate should lessen as healing progresses.
- *Alginate dressing* (e.g. Kaltostat or Sorbsan). The level of exudate will determine the type of dressing required.

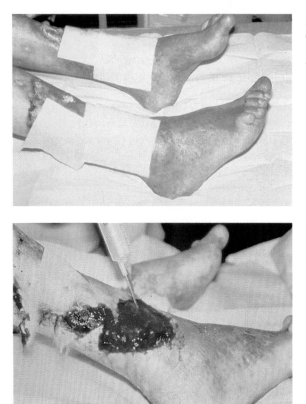

Figure 4.12(a). An alginate dressing, Sorbsan, being applied to a deep, heavily exuding ulcer.

Figure 4.12(b). The dressing is readily removed by irrigation.

4.5.3.6 Sensitivity to wound care products Sensitivity to components found in topical skin and wound preparations is a common phenomenon in patients with leg ulcers (Fraki *et al.*, 1979). Signs and symptoms of a sensitivity reaction include marked erythema of the skin where the product has been in contact, aggravation of pre-existing eczematous conditions and itching.

The most common causes of sensitivity reactions include:

- *Topical antibiotics* (e.g. neomycin or framycetin sulphate).
- *Bases of ointments* (e.g. lanolin).
- *Preservatives* (e.g. parabens).

Several proprietary antiseptics and antihistamine creams that patients buy and administer to themselves can also cause an adverse skin reaction.

The paste bandages (*Table 4.3*) can cause sensitivity reactions in some patients. The longer the ulcer has been open, the more skin and wound care products the patient is likely to be sensitive to.

Figure 4.13(a). Granuflex E hydrocolloid wafer on removal from a heavily exuding ulcer.

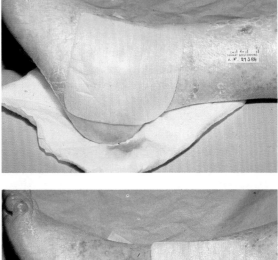

Figure 4.13(b). Minimum handling of the wound bed is necessary, as it is healthily granulating.

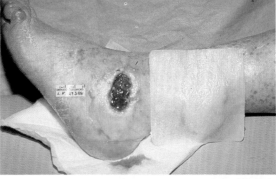

Figure 4.14. A polyurethane foam sheet, Allevyn, being applied to a clean, high exudate ulcer.

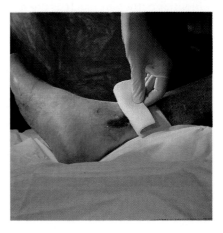

If a sensitivity reaction does occur, use of the sensitizing agent should be discontinued at once and the event clearly documented in the patient's notes. A 1% hydrocortisone cream may be prescribed by the doctor for application only to the skin surrounding the ulcer. Only the blandest of dressings, such as a non-medicated paraffin tulle dressing should be applied to the wound itself.

Patch testing can be helpful in identifying allergens but the results should be viewed with caution. Late positive reactions can occur (Paramsothy *et al.*, 1988) 3 weeks or more after the patch test, and the skin on the back, where patch testing is often performed, is less readily sensitized than the skin surrounding the ulcer, which is why some doctors suggest carrying out the patch test on the same leg instead, a little above the ulcer.

4.5.4 Ultrasound

Several studies have suggested that ultrasound can promote healing in chronic wounds, and results in healed wounds with greater strength and elasticity. Callam *et al.* (1987) found that a once-weekly treatment with ultrasound was effective when used as an adjunct to compression therapy.

4.5.5 Surgical intervention: skin grafting

The healing of large venous ulcers may be rapidly accelerated by simple skin grafting methods, using either pinch (*Figure 4.15*) or meshed split skin. This can even be performed on outpatients taken as day cases, but greater success is likely to be attained with inpatient care. Before grafting is carried out a period of bed rest is usually required to reduce oedema and promote the formation of healthy granulation tissue. The successful take of a graft requires a 'clean' wound bed, free from potential pathogens such as haemolytic streptococci and pseudomonads.

A successful skin graft can give a new lease of life to a patient who has suffered from chronic ulceration for many years (Moody, 1984) but, in itself, is no guarantee that ulceration will not recur.

4.6   Wider issues

4.6.1 Causes of delayed healing

The main cause of delayed healing in leg ulcers is:

FAILURE TO IDENTIFY AND TREAT THE UNDERLYING
CAUSE OF THE ULCER

Other causes of delayed healing include local wound infection (Section 4.5.3.1), sensitivity to wound care products (Section 4.5.3.6) and a number of *general patient factors* (see *Figure 3.5*). Factors particularly significant for patients with leg ulcers include:

- Restricted mobility.
- Oedema in the limb.
- Malnutrition.
- Psychosocial problems.

4.6.2   Restricted mobility

Poor mobility is a common problem for elderly patients with leg ulcers, whether because of joint stiffness, neuromuscular disorders, obesity or respiratory problems. It is essential to improve mobility in patients with any type of leg ulcer. This aids venous return by activating the calf muscle pump, as well as reducing the risk of other problems associated with prolonged immobility such as chest infections and deep vein thromboses.

Patients should be encouraged to mobilize to the limits of their ability. For a patient with advanced arterial disease the limit may be 100–200 yards or metres, or even less. By contrast, many patients with venous ulcers are capable of walking 2–3 miles (3–5 km) per day, and should be encouraged to do so. This is the ideal but may be unattainable for many elderly patients, especially if their poor mobility is accompanied by chronic respiratory problems.

The *physiotherapist* may need to be involved if the patient has restricted ankle movements or other musculoskeletal problems. House-bound patients can be encouraged to walk on the spot for a few minutes every hour. Prolonged standing in one place should be avoided. Washing up and ironing can be done sitting down if chairs of suitable height are available. Chair-bound patients can be taught ankle extension, flexion and rotation exercises by the physiotherapist or nurse.

4.6.3   Peripheral oedema

There are many causes of peripheral oedema including cardiac failure, liver disease, venous disease and malnutrition. Peripheral oedema in a dependent limb can also be encountered in a patient with hemiparesis following a cerebrovascular accident. Identification by the doctor of the underlying cause of the oedema is important, as this will in part determine the treatment.

Whatever its cause, peripheral oedema in the lower limb delays healing by increasing the diffusion distance between blood capillaries and the tissues they serve, so that the tissues become starved of oxygen and nutrients and metabolic waste products build up.

No attempt should be made to reduce oedema by applying compression bandages: this can cause further ischaemia and breakdown of tissues, especially over bony prominences.

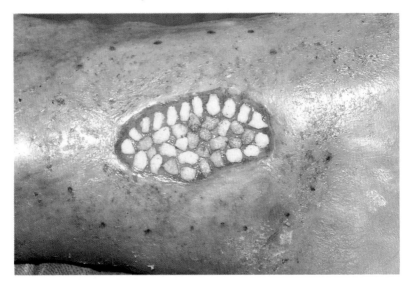

Figure 4.15. Pinch skin grafting.

Improving mobility (see Section 4.6.2) is one very important way of reducing oedema. For patients with venous ulcers, sitting with the legs elevated *above the level of the hips* (*Figure 4.16*) helps to reduce oedema by aiding venous return of blood to the heart. It is *not* sufficient to raise the legs a little above the ground by placing them on a low foot stool. Most patients will benefit from sleeping with the *foot of the bed raised by about 9 inches* (23 cm). This aids venous return and can significantly reduce oedema overnight. However, sudden return of fluid to the heart caused by leg elevation can precipitate cardiac and/or respiratory failure in frail elderly patients. It is therefore advisable to check with the patient's physician that leg elevation is not contraindicated. It is unlikely to be tolerated in patients with poor arterial circulation, who often find it necessary to lower the affected limb below the heart to reduce ischaemic rest pain.

Severe oedema can be alleviated by bed rest, but prolonged bed rest causes problems of its own. Patients may be less mobile when they get up, with stiffened ankle and knee joints. They may develop a chest infection, or a deep vein thrombosis which could further damage the valves in their veins.

4.6.4 Malnutrition
As with all wounds, delayed healing is inevitable if the patient's diet is deficient in protein, calories, vitamins (such as A and C) and minerals (such as iron, zinc and copper).

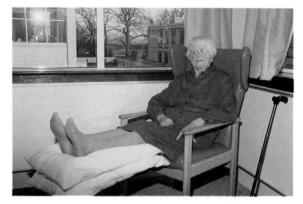

Figure 4.16. Elevation of the legs at rest, above the level of the hips.

Malnutrition is a common problem for the elderly for many reasons: poverty, difficulty in getting to the shops and in preparing food, loss of interest in diet when living alone, and ill-fitting dentures, as well as specific gastrointestinal disorders involving malabsorption problems.

If malnutrition is suspected, a full patient assessment should be carried out by the *dietician* (Goodinson, 1986; Williams, 1986). If the diet is deficient in vitamins and minerals, overweight patients can be just as 'malnourished' as the obviously underweight patient. **The control of obesity can make a crucial contribution to ulcer healing** by reducing prolonged back pressure in the venous system, caused by deep vein obstruction in the pelvic area (see *Figure 2.3*), as well as by enabling increased mobility.

Where the causes of malnutrition are largely social, the *health visitor* or *social worker* can help to arrange meals on wheels, lunch club activities, etc.

4.6.5 Psychosocial issues

Many patients with leg ulcers are elderly, poor and alone. They welcome the visit of the community nurse treating their ulcer because of the social contact that it brings.

Much has been written about the 'social' ulcer. There is no doubt that some patients do not have a vested interest in their ulcer healing, but the proportion of patients who actually *interfere* with the ulcer in an attempt to delay healing is unknown.

Many patients who interfere with their bandages do so for very good reason:

- The bandage may have been applied under *too much tension*, especially over the dorsum of the foot, causing considerable discomfort.
- The bandage may have slipped, causing a tight band of constriction, and pain over a bony prominence.
- A bulky bandage may be causing the patient problems with wearing ordinary footwear.

Prodding a knitting needle between the bandage and the leg may be the patient's solution to an intolerable itch, rather than a wilful attempt at undoing the nurse's good work. The natural recurrence rate for leg ulceration is also high, especially if no measures are taken to prevent recurrence.

If, after exploring with the patient the reasons behind obvious tampering with bandages and dressings, a conscious attempt at self-inflicted injury is still suspected, the problem *must* be dealt with sympathetically. If the problem is one of loneliness, ways of improving the patient's social contacts should be explored with the health visitor or social work department. If the patient is finding it increasingly difficult to cope alone at home, some form of day care may need to be considered.

References

Brennan, S.S., Foster, M. E. and Leaper, D.J. (1986) Antiseptics toxicity in wounds healing by secondary intention. *J. Hosp. Infect.* **8**(3), 263–267.

Callam, M.J., Harper, D.R., Dale, J.J. *et al.* (1987) A controlled trial of weekly ultrasound therapy in chronic leg ulceration. *Lancet* **ii**, 204–206.

Clay, C.S. and Cherry, G.W. (1990) Improvement in skin quality using Granuflex Adhesive Compression Bandage. *Care: Science and Practice* **8**(2), 84–87.

Dale, J.D. and Gibson, B. (1990) Back-up for the venous pump: compression hosiery. *Professional Nurse* **5**(9), 481–486.

Eriksson, G., Eklund, A. and Kallings, L.O. (1984) The clinical significance of bacterial growth in venous leg ulcers. *Scand. J. Infect. Dis.* **16**, 175–180.

Fraki, J.E., Peltonen, L. and Hopsu-Havu, V.K. (1979) Allergy to various components of topical preparations in stasis dermatitis and leg ulcer. *Contact Dermatitis* **5**, 97–100.

Goodinson, S.M. (1986) Assessment of nutritional status. *Nursing* **3**(7), 252–257.

Hazarika, E.Z. and Wright, D.E. (1981) Chronic leg ulcers: the effect of pneumatic intermittent compression. *Practitioner* **225**, 189–192.

Leaper, D.J. and Simpson, R.A. (1986) The effect of antiseptics and topical antimicrobials on wound healing. *J. Antimicrob. Chemother.* **17**(2), 135–137.

Moody, M. (1984) A new lease of life. *Nursing Times* (July 4), 46.

Morison, M.J. (1990) Wound cleansing – which solution? *Nursing Standard* **4**(52), Suppl 4–6.

Morison, M.J. (1991) *The Nursing Management of Wounds.* Austen Cornish, London.

Paramsothy, Y., Collins, M. and Smith, G.M. (1988) Contact dermatitis in patients with leg ulcers: the prevalence of late positive reactions. *Contact Dermatitis* **18**, 30–36.

Sockalingham, S., Barbenel, J.C. and Queen, D. (1990) Ambulatory monitoring of the pressures beneath compression bandages. *Care: Science and Practice* **8**(2), 75–79.

Williams, C.M. (1986) Wound healing: a nutritional perspective. *Nursing* **3**(7), 249–251.

5. *Patient education*

Where patients are truly partners with the health care team in planning their care and monitoring its progress, compliance with treatment and rapid reporting of adverse reactions is most likely.

There are many strategies available for teaching patients (Coutts and Hardy, 1985), including:

- *Videos of bandaging techniques*, for the able patient who is reapplying a heavy compression bandage daily.
- *Group discussions*, for alert patients attending an outpatient clinic.
- *Information leaflets*, on care of legs and other self-help measures, for leg ulcer patients and/or their carers.

An individualized health education programme should be devised, bearing in mind the patient's cognitive abilities and learning needs.

Patient education is an *ongoing process* and should include, where appropriate:

- A simple explanation of the underlying cause of the ulcer.
- Advice on: exercise, reducing oedema, leg care, nutrition, compliance with treatment.

It is important, however, that patients receive certain *key information* at their *first consultation*:

- The nurse's name and workplace.
- A contact phone number.
- The simple signs and symptoms that suggest that treatment may need to be changed quickly, such as increased pain, redness, itching or loss of sensation in the leg.

THIS INFORMATION SHOULD BE WRITTEN DOWN AND LEFT WITH THE PATIENT OR GIVEN TO THE PRINCIPAL CARE GIVER.

Further guidance on patient education in relation to wound management is given in Morison (1991). A example of an information leaflet suitable for patients with venous ulcers and for their carers is given in *Table 5.1.*

Table 5.1 – How to care for your legs (for patients with venous leg ulcers)

How long must I keep the dressing and bandage or (stocking) in place?

Wear the support bandages or elastic support stockings as advised by the doctor and nurse. They will make arrangements for your next dressing change.

Do not be tempted to look under the bandages or disturb the dressing in the meantime as this may delay healing. It is particularly important not to scratch the skin around the ulcer as this skin is easily damaged.

Ask for help at once if:
- Your leg is more itchy, hot or painful than usual.
- You feel that the bandage is too tight anywhere.
- You lose sensation in your toes, they turn cold or blue.
- You need any other advice.

Contact person: ....

Contact telephone number: ....

Can I exercise?

Yes, exercise is good for your circulation and your general health. If possible take a gentle walk every day. Even indoors you can bend and stretch your toes while sitting. Bend, flex, and circle your ankles to prevent them from becoming stiff. It is important not to stand still for too long. It is a good idea to do the dishes and the ironing while sitting down if you can obtain a chair of the correct height.

Should I sit with my legs up?

Yes. Sitting with your legs hanging down is almost as bad as standing in one place for too long. You should sit with your legs elevated above the level of your hips, supported by a stool, a cushion or a pillow. It is also helpful to raise the foot of your bed 9 inches, as this aids return of blood from the legs to the heart.

Do I need a special diet?

You do not need a special diet but try to eat a balanced one that includes protein (meat, fish, eggs), fresh fruit and vegetables. Being overweight does not help the circulation in your legs. Ask the doctor for advice on weight loss if this is a problem for you.

Are there any other ways I can help my legs?
- Avoid knocks to your legs as this could lead to another ulcer.
- Keep your legs warm, but do not sit too close to the fire as this can damage the skin.
- Don't wear anything around the tops of your legs (garters or girdles) as this hinders the circulation.
- Stop smoking.

Reference

Coutts, L.C. and Hardy, L.K. (1985) Teaching for Health: The Nurse as Health Educator. Churchill Livingstone, Edinburgh.

Morison, M.J. (1991) *The Nursing Management of Wounds*. Austen Cornish, London.

6. Preventing recurrence of leg ulceration

The recurrence rate for leg ulceration is very high (see *Table 1.1*). Following the self-help advice given in Section 4.6 and *Table 5.1* should go some way to improving the local conditions in the lower leg. The patient should be advised to avoid knocking the leg but should not be discouraged from going into public places, where such trauma is most likely to occur. Social isolation can be one of the biggest problems for patients with recurring ulcers.

For patients with venous ulcers, wearing compression hosiery (*Figure 6.1*), even after the ulcer has healed (Dale and Gibson, 1990), is probably the best way of preventing recurrence. For some patients, surgery to correct the underlying vascular disorder may be beneficial (Negus and Friegood, 1983).

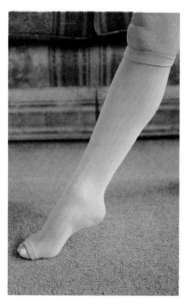

Figure 6.1. A class 2 compression stocking.

References

Dale, J.D. and Gibson, B. (1990) Back-up for the venous pump: compression hosiery. *Professional Nurse* **5**(9), 481–486.

Negus, D. and Friegood, A. (1983) The effective management of venous ulceration. *Br. J. Surg.* **70**, 623–627.

Further reading

Compression bandages and hosiery

Cornwall, J.V., Dore, C.J. and Lewis, J.D. (1987) Graduated compression and its relation to venous refilling time. *British Medical Journal* **295**, 1087–1090.

Dale, J.D. and Gibson, B. (1990) Back-up for the venous pump: compression hosiery. *Professional Nurse* **5**(9), 481–486.

Fentem, P.H. (1990) Defining the compression provided by hosiery and bandages. *Care: Science and Practice* **8**(2), 53–55.

Thomas, S. (1990) Bandages and bandaging. *Nursing Standard* **4**(39), Supplement, 4–6.

The ischaemic leg

Orr, M.M. and McAvoy, B.R. (1987) The ischaemic leg. In Fry, J. and Berry, H.E. (eds) *Surgical problems in Clinical Practice*, pp. 123–135. Edward Arnold, London.

Surgical management of venous disease

Ruckley, C.V. (1988) *A Colour Atlas of Surgical Management of Venous Disease.* Wolfe Medical Publications, London.

Wound dressing and local wound management

Morison, M.J. (1991) *The Nursing Management of Wounds.* Austen Cornish, London.

Index

Index